Harnessing Your Dark Feminine Energy

How to Become a Femme Fatale and Step into Your Divine Power

Elva B. Fagan

© Copyrights 2023 – Elva B. Fagan

All rights reserved.

This book's contents may not be reproduced, duplicated, or transmitted without direct written permission from the author or publisher. No blame or legal responsibility will be held against the publisher or author for any damages, reparations, or monetary loss due to the information contained in this book. Whether directly or indirectly.

Disclaimer Notice:

Please note that the information within this document is for educational and entertainment purposes only. All efforts have been made to present reliable and complete information. However, no warranties of any kind are implied or declared.

Table of Contents

Table of Contents iii

Introduction: The Art of Dark Femininity v

Chapter 1: History of the Femme Fatale 1

Chapter 2: Which Femme Fatale Are You? 7
   Types of femme fatales portrayed in film 12

Chapter 3: Secrets of a True Femme Fatale 20
   Confidence 22
   Uniqueness 23
   Mystery 23
   Intelligence 25
   Detachment 26
   Unpredictability 26

Chapter 4: Habits of a Desirable Femme Fatale 29

Chapter 5: Things Highly Confident Femme Fatales Never Do 36

Chapter 6: Become a Femme Fatale 40

Chapter 7: How to be a Magnetizing Woman 45

Chapter 8: Emotional Skills of High-Value Women 56

Chapter 9: Emotional Needs of Men that Make them Addicted to Women 68

Chapter 10: How to Train Men to Respect You 74

Chapter 11: How to Find a Man that will Spoil You 81

Chapter 12: Feminine Energy Morning Affirmations 86

Femme fatale affirmations to Boost your Confidence.......................... 95

Magnetic Femininity Affirmations 99

Chapter 13: Psychology Tricks to Get What You Want Out of People ... 108

Social tricks for influence 112

Tricks to influence people's behavior 116

Chapter 14: Traits of Women Who Have Activated their Dark Feminine Energy 120

Conclusion 127

Introduction: The Art of Dark Femininity

Some people might think being nice is the only way to be feminine, but dark femininity also has its place. Before we dive in, I want to give a quick warning. This might not be the book for you if you're easily offended or uncomfortable with topics that are sometimes considered manipulative or mean. However, if you're open to exploring different facets of femininity and discovering how they can help you achieve your goals, then keep reading.

Overall, dark femininity is a powerful tool that women can use to achieve their goals. It's not about being mean or manipulative but tapping into your desires and using them to your advantage. By embracing your dark femininity, you can become more confident, assertive, and successful personally and professionally.

First, whether light or dark, femininity is all about playing with desire, but dark femininity does this exceptionally well. Desire can be a double-edged sword, though. So, when I say that dark femininity is about playing with desire, it doesn't always have to be bad. For example, flirting is one way to play with desire and can be playful and easygoing. However, flirting can also get dark quickly.

The first trait of dark femininity is mastering the art of playing with desire. If you've ever flirted to get what you want, then you've tapped into your dark femininity. Flirting is all about sending a signal to get what you want. It can be a powerful tool, especially if you have advantages like pretty privilege or a baby face. For example, I know my smile can be mesmerizing, so I use it to my advantage when flirting.

If flirting isn't your thing, you can tap into your sexual appeal to get what you want. This might sound controversial, but it's another way to embrace your dark femininity. For example, if you need a favor from someone at work, you might dress to accentuate your best features and use your charm to persuade them. However, it's important to be cautious and not abuse this approach.

Another way to tap into your dark femininity is to embrace being a damsel in distress. While some may associate this with light femininity, the psychology behind it is linked to dark femininity. When using your dark femininity, you are calculated and will do whatever it takes to achieve your goals. However, it's important to note that relying on this trait too much can lead to corruption.

Understanding the power of a woman in need is the key to using this trait effectively. Even if you can do something yourself, sometimes allowing someone else to help you can work to your advantage. This tactic won't work if you aren't in tune with your light femininity, as being a damsel in distress requires a certain level of femininity.

Remembering that being clingy differs from being a damsel in distress is important. If you're clingy, you're not tapping into your dark femininity; you're simply being miserable. The goal of being a damsel in distress is to get things done and achieve your desired outcome. It's a tactic that can work like a charm on both men and women, regardless of gender.

While it may seem manipulative, there are positive aspects to dark femininity. It helps to balance out your light femininity, allowing you to be assertive without being a pushover. It also helps you achieve your goals, whether flirting your way into or out of something or being a damsel in distress.

However, using your dark femininity in moderation is important, as overuse can lead to predictability and a loss of charm. It's a trait to be used strategically rather than as a default approach to every situation.

Let's dive into the rudiments of dark femininity!

x

Chapter 1: History of the Femme Fatale

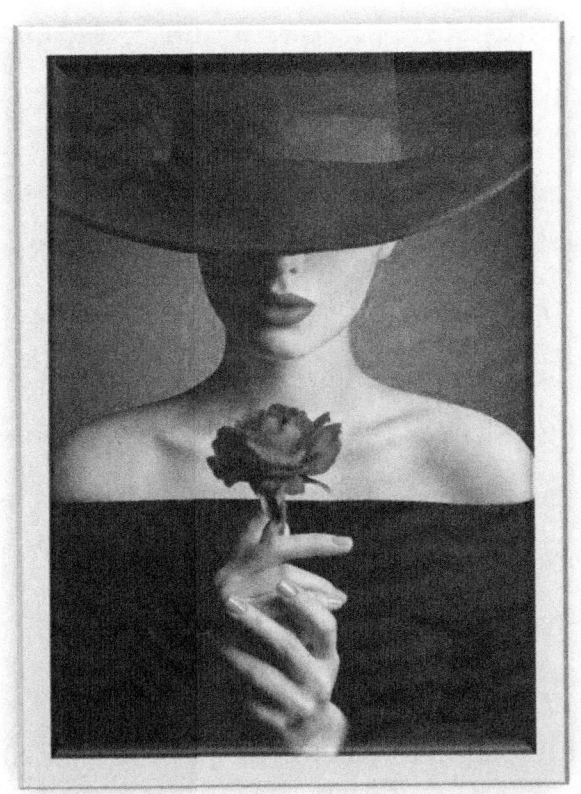

The femme fatale is a character archetype that has existed in various forms throughout literature and media. The Oxford Dictionary defines the femme fatale as "an attractive and seductive woman, especially one who is likely to cause distress or disaster to a man who becomes involved with her." However, many consider this character trope to be anti-feminist, with second-wave feminists, in particular, criticizing its portrayal of women.

The femme fatale is most commonly associated with classic film noir from the 1940s and 1950s, but its roots can be traced back to ancient mythology, including Judeo-Christian and Greek mythologies. For example, Eve from the story of Adam and Eve in the book of Genesis is often considered the first archetypal femme fatale. In Greek mythology, there are also numerous femme fatale figures, such as Medusa, whose beauty and destructive power are intertwined.

The first wave of the femme fatale as a character type emerged in the late 1800s, with male anxieties around rising lower classes, foreign invasion, and feminism influencing depictions of the femme fatale. One reason for anxiety around feminism was the rise in female crime, which was viewed as unnatural. Male violence was understood, but female violence was not. The press regularly registered shock and disgust at the increasing evidence of women killing members of their own families for money, but many of these murderers were actually desperate mothers committing infanticide due to poverty.

While the femme fatale can be seen as problematic in its portrayal of women, it is also a complex and multifaceted archetype that has evolved over time. Its roots in mythology and its portrayal in literature and media reflect larger societal anxieties and preoccupations, particularly around gender and power dynamics.

During the Victorian era, a surge in arsenic poisoning led to the government requiring apothecaries and pharmacists to record all arsenic sales in a poison book. While it is commonly believed that the emergence of the femme fatale in literature and film was due to Victorian men's repression, it is only partially true. Different artistic and literary groups existed in the 19th century, and there was a growing interest in ancient mythologies and esoteric religions, which inspired artists and writers to take inspiration from characters such as Cleopatra, Medusa, and Salome and creatures such as vampires and sirens. This interest may explain why depictions of the 19th-century femme fatale leaned on mystical and orientalist imagery, which Fox Studio later exploited in the 1910s. Theda Bara was the most significant femme fatale actress in early cinema history, who often played this orientalist femme fatale, most notably Cleopatra.

The fall of the femme fatale and the rise of the all-American good girl portrayed by actresses such as Mary Pickford and Clara Beau coincided with the strengthening of anti-immigrant values. Film noir, a genre characterized by a paranoid, claustrophobic, and hopeless worldview, a male protagonist, criminality, lack of morality, and ambiguous plot, became popular after World War II. The visual style conveyed this mood through expressive use of darkness, both real, in predominantly under-lit and night time scenes, and psychologically, through shadows and claustrophobic compositions. The feelings of loss and alienation expressed by the characters in film noir can be seen as the product of the post-war depression and the reorganization of the American economy.

One clear example of this is the film "Mildred Pierce," which came out in 1945. The main character Mildred played by Joan Crawford, becomes a business mogul after leaving her husband and needing to support her daughters. The image of Mildred in a masculine dress style, holding her account books and looking away from her lover typifies this kind of displacement. In general, an aura of uncertainty permeates throughout the film, which can also be seen as an indirect response to the changing dynamics of the traditional family unit due to the introduction of women into the labor force.

The femme fatale is often characterized by a cigarette, long, sexy legs that often dominate the frame, thick luscious lips, and gorgeous wavy hair that frames her face perfectly. And attire that is often very flashy, such as fur shawls and coats, long gloves that extend to the elbows, evening gowns that shimmer and sparkle, clothing that reveals legs, cleavage, arms, back, and/or shoulders, and a sexy pair of high heels. Some scholars view the femme fatale as a manifestation of the male protagonist's internal fears of sexuality and his need to control and repress it.

However, even though the femme fatale trope can be limiting, it can also represent empowerment for women.

Chapter 2: Which Femme Fatale Are You?

In this section, we will explore the Femme Fatale character trope, its origins, and the different types portrayed in film. The term 'Femme Fatale' comes from a French phrase meaning "Deadly Woman" or "lethal woman." It refers to an attractive and seductive woman who can cause distress or disaster to a man who becomes involved with her. This archetype exists in many cultures, folklores, and mystical worlds, where they are referred to as an enchantress, a witch, man-eaters, Vamps, seductress, Tetris, sirens, or charmers.

In film, Femme Fatales are stock characters or archetypes of beautiful women who are seductive and mysterious. They use their charm and feminine energy to entrap their lovers, often leading them into compromising and deadly situations. They are known for their prowess and their ability to enchant and have power over men. Femme Fatales are typically villainous or at least morally ambiguous and always associated with a sense of mystification and unease.

Biblical references also associate women with the Femme Fatale archetype. Some people equate Eve in the Bible as a Femme Fatale due to her influence over Adam. Delilah was bribed to figure out the strengths of the powerful Samson so that she could cut off his hair to weaken him. Jezebel, linked to the phrase "fallen" or "abandoned woman," was perceived to use seduction and manipulation to lure or mislead others into idolatry, heresy, and immorality.

Historically, Cleopatra is another known figure associated with being a Femme Fatale. She was known for her decisive leadership and control over men who would fall to her feet. Julius Caesar and Mark Anthony's obsession with her led to the fall of the Roman Empire. In Greek mythology, Clytemnestra is said to be one of the most notorious Femme Fatales because she plotted and avenged her daughter's death by taking out her husband. Other famous Femme Fatales in history are Marie Antoinette and Hedda Gabler, a character from a play written by Henrik Ibsen who was willful and narcissistic to get what she wanted at the expense of manipulating her husband and friends.

The idea of the unbridled, unrestrained, or uncontrolled liberated woman who uses her femininity to advance or to keep her power trickles down into the 1940s and 50s when we have the film noir era. Film Noir is a French cinematic term that primarily describes stylish Hollywood crime dramas. These films had a low-key post-World War II backdrop and a black-and-white visual style. The stories and attitude of the

Great Depression influenced them. The 1940s and 50s were regarded as the classic period in American film Noir. In these films, there is usually a detective or a private eye type figure who is investigating a crime by some law-abiding citizen who's lured into a life of crime or a victim of circumstance. Inside this film style, you will see other genres such as your old classic gangster films, procedurals, Gothic romance, and social issues. And the most memorable stock character, the Femme Fatale, is the intelligent, mysterious, and seductive woman who seems to be tied to the plot and the thick of it all, which is why these characters are so compelling.

During World War II, men were sent off to fight, and women were called upon to work in factories and help create war equipment to aid the war effort. This was a turning point for women, as they could work and be independent for one of the first times in history. This newfound empowerment and female ambition led to the rise of the Riveter campaign, featuring the image of a woman in overalls flexing her muscles. However, this caused paranoia in men who believed women had gained too much power and independence and were no longer interested in being mothers and homemakers. This caused gender roles to become unbalanced and was very scary for men, leading to post-war discomfort.

Upon returning home from war, soldiers began to question and worry that their wives or girlfriends may have been unfaithful to them while they were away overseas, causing them to obsess over female fidelity. They were anxious that women were now unleashed and unhinged, wanting everything to be the same as when they left: the woman inside the home or the men outside working. But instead, they were faced with the newly liberated woman who wanted to continue her newfound freedom. This caused many conflicts between couples, even if the woman had been faithful. The film industry capitalized on this moment, with movies like Gilda featuring themes of perception versus reality or imagination versus reality.

Types of femme fatales portrayed in film

The role of women during World War II and the subsequent societal changes caused by their newfound independence led to the rise of the femme fatale archetype in film. Each type of femme fatale portrayed in film reflects different aspects of society's attitudes towards women, including their sexuality, ambition, and materialism.

When it comes to portraying women in movies, the femme fatale is a well-known archetype that has been present for decades. While the concept of the femme fatale has evolved, it remains a popular and intriguing character type.

We will explain the different femme fatale types that has been portrayed in films below.

The misrepresented femme fatale

This type is deemed sneaky or untrustworthy, manipulative, or falsely accused of using her body or looks to get what she wants based solely on her appearance. This woman is usually innocent and does not have any ill intent while still understanding the power that her beauty and femininity possess. They like to look and feel sexy but may be punished for it and are often associated with distrust, and are usually redeemed in the end.

The ambitious career woman

This femme fatale type can do anything to protect what she loves. She does not want to be restricted to gender roles and takes pride in their independence. They have a need and a will to create success and will do what it takes to get it. However, this type is usually driven by a weakness, which acts as their Kryptonite, causing them to protect this particular weakness fiercely and sometimes blindly. Cersei from 'Game of

Thrones' is a good example of this type, as she was ruthless when protecting her children.

The materialistic femme fatale

This femme fatale type loves wealth, wants the finer things in life, and will do anything to get it. This type is well aware of her beauty and charisma and their effect on others and will use it to her advantage to maintain privilege or what is considered the good life. An example of this type is Veda Pierce, Mildred Pierce's daughter in the film Mildred Pierce, who manipulates, lies, blackmails, and even has an affair with her mother's husband to maintain her lavish lifestyle. She was ruthless in pursuing material wealth and status, even if it meant betraying her mother.

The vengeful femme fatale

This type is usually a woman who was good and honest at first but was poorly treated or taken advantage of by people and society in a way that was not justified. This causes her to have a cynical view of the world and seek revenge. These women use their femininity as a weapon, much like a rebel with a cause. Examples of this type include Faye Dunaway's character in "Chinatown," Carrie Mulligan's character in "Promising Young Woman," and Amy in "Gone Girl."

The literal femme fatale

This femme fatale type is also known as the man-eater. This type is seen in characters like Megan Fox's character in "Jennifer's Body" and the robots in "Ex Machina."

The bored housewife

This type is the bored housewife or woman who wants to escape societal pressures. These women feel controlled and overlooked by their husbands and are unhappy and frustrated in their marriage and place in life. They will do anything to escape their situation, such as Phyllis Dietrichson in "Double Indemnity" and the women in "The Stepford Wives."

The faded beauty

This type is driven by her beauty and was used to getting what she wanted, but she is now older and fearful that her beauty will fade, not yielding the advantages and privileges she had when she was younger and beautiful. Examples include Norma Desmond in "Sunset Boulevard."

The psychological gamer

This type is beyond ruthless and loves psychoanalytical mind games. They are mental giants, very cerebral, smart, cold, and calculating. Examples include Sharon Stone's character Catherine Trammell in "Basic Instinct."

The real-life femme fatale

These women are confident, beautiful, and magnetic. They are capable, independent and aware of their effect on others. They can positively use this power and have a strong presence and feminine energy.

These different types of femme fatales have unique traits and motivations but share a common thread of being powerful and intriguing characters. However, some people find this trope troubling for various reasons. Some see it as misogynistic because the Femme Fatale can denote the notion that women need to be tamed or reined in. They argue that a woman who is liberated or exerts too much feminine energy is seen as dangerous, promiscuous, and toxic, making them a formidable opponent to their male counterparts. On the other hand, some see the Femme Fatale as too feminist, stating that it's anti-men and emasculates them. Some people view them as both.

Another theory is that the Femme Fatale Trope was inserted into movies as a reminder of why gender roles are important and that the Femme Fatale represents what happens when they are not.

Despite these criticisms, the Femme Fatale remains a popular and intriguing character. People are drawn to them for the same reason they are attracted to the bad boy type; they are exciting and have an element of danger that keeps you interested. It's like riding a roller coaster; the adrenaline rush is irresistible.

Femme Fatales have an allure that makes people feel alive. They are different, unique, and possess both beauty and brains, which makes them hypnotic because they intrigue you both physically and mentally. They are like human chess pieces; clever and masterful. Although sometimes they use their strengths for bad, they are fun to watch. It's intriguing to see how these characters take power and how they can turn a good guy and open him to his dark side or awaken something inside of him that he didn't even know existed.

Femme Fatales are masterminds, and who doesn't love watching a brilliant mind at work?

Although you don't want to fall victim to them, they are so irresistible because they show the crux of what it means to be human. They display the good and the bad traits and remind us of our vulnerabilities, temptations, and the most dormant hidden sides of us that can be awakened with the right person under the right circumstances at any moment.

Chapter 3: Secrets of a True Femme Fatale

Have you ever noticed how some women have a magnetic presence, shifting the energy when they enter a room? Despite being a man's Kryptonite, men are still drawn to them. In this section, we'll explore the characteristics of a true Femme Fatale in the modern-day and whether they are masterminds or manipulators. We'll also discuss how to use these traits to your advantage and become irresistible.

Many people have misconceptions about Femme Fatales. Some think it's all about seduction or appearance, but it's more complicated than that. Some people base their knowledge on movies or hearsay, but others have experience and deep analysis of the topic.

So, what is a Femme Fatale?

The term comes from the French meaning of fatal woman or lethal woman. These women are attractive, seductive, and often villainous or morally ambiguous in film. They use their charm to entrap their lovers, leading them into deadly situations. In real life, a Femme Fatale is someone with an innate, inherited, and intuitive way of being. It's a mindset and way of being that comes naturally or can be adopted with time. Confidence is key; it takes natural ability, time, craft, and skill to develop such confidence.

These qualities combined make Femme Fatales a force to be reckoned with. They are smart, cunning, and know how to get what they want. So, it's best to understand them first before trying to outsmart them.

Let's now dive into the key characteristics of a true Femme Fatale.

Confidence

First, they are confident and can hold their own. They are big on self-care and understanding what makes them attractive to others. They care for their inner and outer appearance and know what clothing accentuates their curves and best features. They are clean, polished, and aesthetically pleasing to be around. They capitalize on areas that other women may slack on and are usually not jealous or inferior to other women. Femme Fatales love challenges and take pride in their individuality, rocking to the beat of their own drum. They don't worry about what others are doing but focus on what works best for them.

Becoming a Femme Fatale takes time, effort, and confidence. It's not about seduction or appearance but rather a way of being that comes naturally or can be developed. By embodying the key characteristics of a Femme Fatale, you, too, can have a magnetic presence and become irresistible.

Uniqueness

These women express their individuality through clothing and accessories, carefully selecting the right colors and styles to suit each occasion. They know when to wear red or how to use it as a pop color, and they are not afraid to experiment to add a touch of edge to their look. They don't mind being the center of attention, and they understand the power of their uniqueness to make others wonder and admire them.

Mystery

At the same time, they always leave something to the imagination, preferring to keep an air of mystery around themselves. They understand the importance of balance and give and take, and they won't reveal everything at once. They like to maintain a sense of power and control and won't make big announcements until they are sure of their success. They are naturally private people and understand that moving in silence is often better than making a lot of noise.

These women know their worth and position themselves to win and be successful. They understand the power of elegance and balance and won't show too much of any one body part, preferring to cover up in other areas. They don't have to be the loudest voice in the room, but when they speak, others listen, and men are interested in what they say. They don't come across as nagging or overly thirsty, which makes them even more intriguing.

In contrast, women who reveal everything may excite men temporarily, but they can quickly become boring because there is nothing left to wonder about. These women understand the power of leaving something to the imagination and appreciate it when others work a little harder to get to know them. They are naturally mysterious, and this makes them all the more attractive.

Intelligence

Intelligence is a key quality necessary for them to do what they do. These women are very cerebral, capable, and whip-smart. They are thinkers who like to calculate their moves carefully and avoid errors. They like to think things through to know how to react in most situations. They are very good at understanding their strengths and weaknesses and know how to manipulate people to get what they want.

Manipulation is a trait they possess and can use for good or bad, depending on the situation. They are usually quiet and observant, studying people to know how to work them if needed. They are masters of slinking, which means that they know how to move quietly and unobtrusively. This is an underrated quality of a Femme fatale, and they use it to their advantage to tease and intrigue others.

Detachment

Femme Fatales also understand the power of detachment. They play cat-and-mouse games and avoid getting too attached to anything or anyone without a solid return on investment. They give healthy doses of attention and then pull back to keep others interested. They know when to leave and are not afraid to do so to protect themselves.

Unpredictability

Femme fatales have certain innate qualities that make them irresistible. One of these qualities is unpredictability. When you're unpredictable, people become curious and want to know more about you. You can be unpredictable in many ways, such as speaking in a way that's unexpected of you or changing up your appearance. A femme fatale may appear conservative during the day but reveal a more seductive side at night. The key is to have a sense of humor, always have an unexpected comeback, be enthusiastic, and enjoy being present.

Another quality of a femme fatale is their understanding of the power of feminine energy. They know that it's not just about putting on a revealing outfit but about showing just enough to be a tease. They understand what works for their body and what flatters them. They exude sexiness from within and have an attitude that breeds confidence. They know how to use their body language, such as how they look at a man, enter or exit a room, and smile.

Femme fatales are intentional. They know what they want, when they want it, and how they will get it. They plan ahead and have backup plans. Thinking ahead makes them feel safe and comfortable. They don't waste their time or energy on things that don't serve them.

If you want to embody the qualities of a femme fatale, you need to have self-confidence, believe in yourself, be intentional, and know what you want. By doing so, you'll be powerful and irresistible.

Chapter 4: Habits of a Desirable Femme Fatale

The femme fatale character is a truly iconic figure, exuding confidence, seduction, femininity, and style. In this chapter, we'll explore some of the habits of a femme fatale that we can incorporate into our daily lives. If you want to transform yourself into a highly desirable, seductive, and irresistible woman, then keep on reading.

Put yourself first

When we think of a femme fatale, we envision a woman who prioritizes herself above everything else. This is because she knows that the best investment she can make is in herself. Investing in your wardrobe, beauty routine, hair, fitness, environment, and overall well-being is crucial to becoming the best version of yourself. So, let's all take a page from the femme fatale's book and start prioritizing ourselves.

The femme fatale has a unique mindset and approach to life. One of her top priorities is investing in herself. Although she enjoys the finer things in life, she doesn't rely solely on her husband for financial support. The femme fatale knows that putting herself first isn't a selfish act. It means prioritizing her goals and desires above everything else without using or being mean to others. This attitude makes the femme fatale a force to be reckoned with.

Sometimes, pursuing one's goals means letting go of certain people. But the femme fatale accepts this as a part of life and believes there's a season for everything. She understands that leveling up is about taking care of oneself and becoming the best version of oneself. This mentality is what sets the femme fatale apart.

When it comes to fashion, the femme fatale wears whatever makes her feel fabulous. She's always glamorous, beautiful, and put together. Whether it's red, black, or any other color, she loves to wear dresses that show off her figure. Jewelry is also a must-have for the femme fatale. She never lets other people's opinions or judgments affect her style choices. Instead, she focuses on building her confidence by daring to wear what she wants.

Positive thinking

Being a confident woman in today's society is not easy – the femme fatale knows this all too well. People may stare or comment, but she focuses on positive thoughts about herself. She believes having a positive mindset is the key to not caring about other people's opinions. Remembering that people's looks don't always signify negative thoughts is essential. Thinking positively about oneself is always better and helps in building confidence. Ultimately, the femme fatale encourages others to stay positive, focus on their goals and desires, and wear whatever makes them feel fabulous.

When we think of a femme fatale, certain characteristics come to mind, such as a specific look, aura, confidence, and way of carrying herself. However, there is one more important trait that is often overlooked, which is her intoxicating perfume. A femme fatale chooses a specific perfume that represents her, and when she's walking around, you recognize it, and you recognize that it's her. So, choosing a beautiful perfume that represents you and makes you feel feminine, attractive, and confident is important. This will be your signature perfume, and it can make you feel sexy and fabulous.

Unpredictability

Another characteristic of a femme fatale is her unpredictability. While it's important to be someone others can count on, sometimes it's fun to add a little spice and be unpredictable. A femme fatale is extremely mysterious, and her mystery is about unpredictability. You never know what she will do next, which creates attraction and allure. Men love this type of energy because it's exciting and alluring.

So, how can you be more unpredictable like a femme fatale?

You can change your habits, your look, or even your mind. Being more spontaneous can add a touch of spice and mystery to your personality.

We don't have to be one-dimensional women. We can be many different things, including a sensual femme fatale. By choosing the right perfume and being more unpredictable, we can add a touch of allure and mystery to our personality, which is an important part of our femininity. So, embrace your inner femme fatale and let your unpredictable and intoxicating energy shine.

Her presence is expensive

It's not just about her luxurious taste and good quality clothes. It's about her aura and how she makes you feel lucky to be in her presence. She's not always available, which makes her presence even more valuable. If you want to make your presence expensive, focus on your aura, confidence, and how you carry yourself rather than just looking expensive. When you know your worth and what you want and don't want and embody those desires naturally, you exude a powerful energy that draws people toward you.

The woman who embodies all these qualities is also mysterious, passionate, exciting, and enticing. She doesn't reveal everything or her next move, which only adds to her allure. Mystery is attractive because it makes people want to possess something they can't have. She can protect and execute her plans without interference by moving in silence.

Overall, the woman with an expensive presence exudes confidence and embodies her desires naturally. She knows her worth and what she wants, and her mysterious aura only adds to her attractiveness.

Chapter 5: Things Highly Confident Femme Fatales Never Do

Femme fatales are excellent examples of confidence and how to hold oneself to a certain standard.

Firstly, she never looks bad. Regardless of the situation, she always looks glamorous and put together, often overdressed but never out of place. She takes care of herself and makes a stunning first impression wherever she goes. Even at home, she lounges in beautiful and glamorous nightgowns.

Secondly, a confident femme fatale always smells fantastic. She has a timeless taste in perfume and fashion, often preferring dark colors and luxurious textures like silk, velvet, and faux fur. She is not one to chase trends, instead opting for a classic and elegant style with a touch of sensuality.

A confident femme fatale always looks good, smells good, and exudes magnetic charisma and feminine power. She is an excellent example of how to hold oneself to a high standard while embracing elegance and glamour.

She never compromises her boundaries, standards, and values. She does not allow anyone to downgrade her, and she eliminates people from her life who do not respect her. This is because she is confident in herself and her worth and does not need validation from others.

Additionally, the femme fatale is never desperate. She has an abundance mindset and knows everything she desires will come to her. She is not clingy or needy and lets others know she is desirable and valuable. This makes her an irresistible challenge and adds to her allure.

While the femme fatale may be independent and not a people pleaser, she is still elegant, considerate, and loving towards those she cares about.

The femme fatale is elegant with high emotional intelligence, evident in how she controls her emotions. She doesn't lash out in front of others when angry and knows when it's not the right time to do so. This level of maturity is attractive and important to many people. The femme fatale is also sociable, gifted in discussion, and never treat others as if they are below her. She exudes charm and charisma, and while she may be playful and sarcastic, she never hurts or criticizes others. She is highly confident and doesn't need to put others down to feel good about herself. The femme fatale values people and ignores those who don't deserve her time. She loves the finer things in life but is discreet and private about her possessions and money, as she believes that arrogance is not charming but rather a sign of desperation. The femme fatale exudes energy and the essence of confidence, self-love, and being unbothered.

In summary, the femme fatale is a confident, unique individual who celebrates other women, is true to herself, maintains her privacy, and does not let emotions rule her life. These qualities make her a powerful and fascinating presence in the world.

Chapter 6: Become a Femme Fatale

As a woman, you hold immense power over men, and it's mind-blowing that not all women take advantage of it. Simply by being attractive, taking care of your appearance, and having a bit of a brain, you can seduce men and get almost anything you want. However, it's important to note that there's more to it than just being good-looking. You need to have something about you, a certain persona that attracts men. It's not difficult to figure out how to create this persona. You can learn by observing women who inspire you and imitating their behavior. Don't copy everything about them; learn from what makes them attractive.

Being a woman today is truly a privilege. Despite some challenges that come with the territory, such as pregnancy and periods, women today have the freedom to cheat on their partners if mistreated or cheated on. Men often remarry women with children from multiple partners, regardless of their age or situation. So, if you're a woman, you're in luck. Ignore people who try to discourage you by telling you that you won't find a partner because of your age or the number of children you have. The truth is people will make their own decisions regardless of how many warnings they receive.

So, don't waste time listening to things that bring you down. Look at the real world and see how women are getting remarried all the time, no matter their age, situation, or number of children. The world is full of crazy people, and men marry them too. Focus on creating an attractive persona and taking advantage of your power as a woman.

Being a woman has many advantages, and today, women have more opportunities than ever before. However, some men still hold outdated beliefs about women, such as the idea that younger women are more desirable than older ones. Being a good-looking woman can give you many opportunities, but it's important to use your brain and have a strategy to make the most of these opportunities.

In today's world, any woman at any age can be good-looking and get whatever she desires. Men are aware of this fact, and it's something that they are envious of. So, why aren't more women taking advantage of this? Life is short, so why not experience what it's like to be treated like a goddess?

It's also incredible how much power women hold over men. We can literally sell anything, even things like pictures of our feet or jars of our farts, and men will pay for it. We can also get into clubs for free, and men come to these establishments specifically for women.

However, what's baffling is that not enough women realize the power that they hold. If more women understood the extent of their influence, they wouldn't waste their time with men who have nothing to offer. Men will go to great lengths to obtain the power that women have between their legs.

Women should use their power to their advantage and take control of their lives. It's time for more women to realize their worth and not settle for anything less.

Men and women are biologically different, leading to different advantages and disadvantages in life. Men are often driven by their hormonal desires for sex, which can sometimes cause them to put up with unpleasant situations to pursue a sexual relationship with a woman. In contrast, women have the power to decide when and with whom they want to engage in sexual activity.

Furthermore, women can use their tears to elicit sympathy from others, whereas men who cry are often viewed as weak. Women may also receive more lenient punishments for crimes compared to men, particularly if they are attractive. These advantages can be particularly pronounced for conventionally beautiful women.

In summary, while men and women have different advantages and disadvantages in life, conventionally attractive women can often use this to their advantage in various ways. However, this does not mean women do not face unique pressures and challenges.

Chapter 7: How to be a Magnetizing Woman

Charm is a confusing and perplexing concept for many people. While many can recognize when they have been charmed by someone, they may struggle to articulate what charm is. The reason for this confusion is that charm is not a measurable or palpable quality; instead, it is an aura that emanates from a person. In other words, it is an invisible energy that radiates from a person.

So, what exactly is charm, and what makes a person charming?

Are people born with it, or can a person develop the skill of being charming? And if so, how can you become more charming?

Let's start with the dictionary definition. Charm is defined as the power or quality of lighting, attracting or fascinating others. It is derived from the Latin word "carmen," which means a song, a verse, or an incantation, all closely related to casting a magical spell.

In the context of dating and relationships, charm is seduction without having sex or seduction through the mind only. It is the alchemy of all the non-sexual attributes and attitudes of a person that can capture a person's mind in an obsessive, addictive, and even intoxicating way. In an increasingly rational world where women are more in their masculine energy, therefore less feminine and less charming, men crave to be charmed and fascinated by a woman more than ever before. Yet, it is something they encounter very rarely. This is why being charming and magnetizing is an important tool to add to your arsenal and will give you an edge over other women.

The good news is that charm is not something you are born with or can never have. Being charming is a learned behavior and a skill that can be acquired anytime. Many women develop that skill by observing other charming people in action or reading books like this.

Now, let's discuss how you can become more charming and magnetizing as a woman.

<u>Develop the art of listening</u>

A charming woman listens more than she speaks. She is a master in the art of listening. So, if you want to be charming, you need to learn how to get out of your head and place all of your attention on the other person. When you choose to listen to a man more than you speak about yourself, you send him a signal that you do care about what he has to say. And you also give him space to reveal himself to you and a chance for you to observe and learn more about him while remaining a mystery by not revealing too much about yourself. In other words, you give him the experience of feeling seen and heard, and trust me, it is not something he comes across that often because most people don't really want to listen to anyone, and most people don't care.

Once you learn more about him, it becomes easier to use well-placed and subtle flattery here and there, increasing your likability, but please be genuine when doing so. People and men are no different, love talking about themselves, so if you offer them the space to do it, they will attribute the positive emotion from talking about themselves to you and will associate you with positive emotions. Also, men who tend to evolve in more masculine environments rarely feel seen and heard, so when a woman gives them that experience of feeling seen and heard, she becomes memorable.

Be a source of pleasure

A charming woman is always associated with fun and pleasure and away from drama and problems because, in the imagination of men, a charming woman is not real or ordinary. She embodies the perfect woman fantasy and does not have ordinary people's problems. Of course, this is not true, as there is no such person, but a charming person understands that she does not need to be herself or to be real.

Seducers enjoy performing and are not weighed down by their identity or by some need to be themselves or natural. A charming woman can be pleasant by avoiding bringing her issues, problems, or serious topics into the conversation. This is particularly important when you are just getting to know a man. People, in general, and men, in particular, do not really want to hear about your problems, especially early in their relationship. It triggers negative emotions and reminds them of their own problems that they are attempting to escape in your company, so they subconsciously associate the resultant negative emotions with you and may want to avoid your company in the future.

To be a charming woman, you must aim to be pleasant on many levels. Pleasant to the eye by making an effort to look your absolute best, pleasant to other senses like smelling good, so always wear perfume because your smell leaves a mark on people's minds, and be fun, joyful, and happy. Avoid talking about your work-related and family problems. Also, avoid controversial topics and focus on light and fun conversations.

Adopt feminine body language

Certain body language cues are considered more feminine than others. If you want to exude charm and femininity, it's important to practice and adopt these cues until they become second nature to you.

Start with a beautiful smile – it's a powerful tool that can't be denied. Make sure to smile when conversing with the man you want to charm. Also, maintain good posture by strengthening your back, pulling your shoulders, and elongating your neck. Practice moving gracefully and making gentle movements when picking up or carrying objects like a glass or a bag.

Don't forget to work on your voice and speech, too – slow down your speech and keep your volume low. When it comes to your appearance, choose clothes that flatter your curves and complement your skin tone. Finally, don't be afraid to showcase your feminine and sensual areas, like your neck, by putting your hair up and exposing your shoulders – just be sure not to overdo it.

Be vulnerable

Beauty lies in imperfection and vulnerability. Sharing a well-placed sign of vulnerability can be incredibly charming to a man. It's important to become comfortable sharing insecurities and past scars, but only those you have completely overcome. This is why doing inner work to overcome your issues is crucial. Vulnerability conveys pain, which can create a strong bond between people. By sharing your vulnerability, you'll appear more human and relatable to the man you're interested in. It also reveals the depth of your character and shows that there is more to you than meets the eye. Only those confident enough to live with their insecurities are brave enough to share them. This type of confidence expressed through vulnerability is incredibly charming.

Calmness and self-possession

Calmness and self-possession are important qualities of a charming woman. In our modern society, people lack these qualities because they are always busy running around, pursuing things, and having too much on their plates. Therefore, it is natural to be charmed by a very calm person who gives us a sense of peacefulness and quietness. A charming woman is never in a hurry. She is always composed and rarely shows impatience. She rarely loses her temper, either. She exudes calm, composed, and peaceful energy.

The art of subtlety

Subtlety is the art of indirectly conveying ideas, opinions, or feelings using imagery, metaphors, or other figures of speech. To be a charming woman, you must master the art of subtlety because a charming woman avoids directness and uses indirect suggestions instead. She also uses insinuations by playing with words to convey her message. She uses silence combined with fine gestures to express her opinion. For example, if a man asks her if she wants to do something or go somewhere and her answer is no, a charming woman would avoid saying no directly. She would look at the man, smile, and let the silence speak for her.

Flattering a man's ego through his weaknesses

Every man has insecurities, and a man's ego builds walls to protect those insecurities from being exposed but also seeks anything that would validate him. For men, in particular, a certain level of self-esteem and ego boost is attached to getting a woman's validation. If you become the woman who gives him the validation he craves, he will become addicted to you. Flattering a man based on his weaknesses, such as his vanity or his need to be right, can make you a very addictive and charming woman to him. For example, if he fears not being strong enough, tell him you feel safe with him. If he doubts his sex appeal, tell him you find him attractive. Tell him how intelligent you find him to be if he is the intellectual type. This is a powerful way to penetrate a man's defenses and create surrender.

Be unavailable sometimes

A charming person is somewhat of an illusion, someone who cannot be captured and is a little unpredictable. Therefore, it is important to give a sense of unpredictability and unreliability. A charming woman is not always available, and a man does not always know where she is or what she is doing. Being unavailable sometimes will make his desire for you more intense because there is something charming and appealing about someone who presents challenges.

<u>Be mysterious</u>

A charming woman must have some mystery to her. She cannot be too readable, obvious, present, trivial, or ordinary. A man is charmed when he cannot quite figure out who he is dealing with and cannot put that woman in a box.

Chapter 8: Emotional Skills of High-Value Women

The number one thing that separates high-value women from the rest of women is emotional mastery. So many women were programmed in such a way, not realizing that their success in their romantic life would come down to how well they handle their emotions. So, in this chapter, we will be talking about the emotional skills that I identified as the key skills a woman must possess to achieve emotional mastery and be a high-value woman. This is a vital topic if you experience uncontrollable impulses, mood swings, and negative emotions such as fear, anxiety, anger, hatred, and jealousy. Or if you tend to be volatile, easily affected by other people's opinion of you, or if your well-being depends on other people's behavior towards you, etc.

Self-awareness

The first skill you need to develop to have emotional mastery is self-awareness, and this is the mother of all the other skills because you cannot control what you're not aware of.

Unconscious people interpret situations through the veil of their mental and emotional conditioning. Their lack of awareness of this conditioning makes them unable to differentiate between what is and their own interpretation. Only when they become more aware of their emotional and mental conditioning can they see things for what they really are because they are then able to separate their perception of things and the unbiased reality of things. Therefore, they can have a more realistic assessment of any given situation.

By simply being more aware of your conditioning, your actions no longer have to be dictated by emotional or mental state but instead can be based on an unfiltered and more accurate perception of reality. In other words, through developing awareness, you can control your actions despite your emotional state.

You can work on your self-awareness in many ways, but what I found to be very useful in my own experience is self-reflection and the practice of silence. Practice in silence allows space for you to hear the whisper of your emotions, and the more silence you practice, the louder your emotions become and the more aware you become of them.

You can make a weekly or daily practice of sitting in a quiet room by yourself for 30 minutes and allowing yourself to notice what is happening inside you. Day after day, you will start noticing how you feel, and you may even feel some emotions for things that happened long ago.

Self-reflection is the other practice I found very useful for self-awareness. Again, I would sit down in a quiet room, or I would go to a coffee shop alone, and I would reflect on past events, especially those that caused me a lot of pain, triggered me, made me lose control, or induced a lot of intense emotions in me. Often, I take notes of how I feel as I reflect, and I reverse engineer what caused me to feel the way I did. Then, I go back to my notes every now and then and then reflect on them.

Embrace all your emotions

A high-value woman embraces all her emotions. In other words, there are no right or wrong emotions for a high-value woman. All emotions, good or bad, are accepted because a high-value woman knows that all emotions have a valid reason to be and that every emotion must be listened to because it is trying to tell her something about what is happening inside her. Therefore, instead of being judgmental or dismissive of her emotions, a high-value woman is curious. If she feels negative emotions such as hatred, jealousy, insecurity, etc., she does not suppress them, dismiss them, ignore them, or let them be.

Instead, she asks herself:

Why am I feeling this?

What is it about me or about the situation that induced that particular emotion?

You must learn to embrace all your emotions and use them to learn deeply about yourself if you want to become a high-value woman.

Don't act on your emotions

Accepting your emotions does not mean deciding what to do based on your feelings and letting your emotions run the show. If you look back at some of the mistakes and wrong decisions you made that led to negative consequences in your life, you will find that a lot of them were mainly driven by an intense emotional state you were in at the time that overtook your mind and your rational thinking and prevented you from assessing your options properly.

Using your emotions as the primary input to your decisions can lead to being impulsive and jumping onto situations that are not good for you, or avoiding trying new things that could benefit you out of fear of the unknown, for example. So, it is crucial to be aware that emotions are to be felt, not acted on because they often lead to misconceptions and inadequate actions. Emotions are very useful for self-development purposes. They tell you important things about you, your values, your past traumas, and your programming, and that kind of insight can be used to work on yourself and improve yourself. But when making decisions, a high-value woman always uses logic and intuition, which is very different from emotions.

Have empathy

Empathy is a crucial emotional skill to develop for a high-value woman. It is the ability to see the world through other people's eyes, which helps understand others. It helps connect with others, show compassion, make good social choices, and ultimately develop lasting relationships. It is an emotional skill because it's only when you can understand how the other person feels that you can understand their perspective and respond to them adequately. It is also very useful when uncovering a person's true feelings and intentions and identifying those with harmful intentions.

For example, through her empathy, a high-value woman can spot liars, players, and manipulators no matter how hard they try to hide their bad intentions. It is almost instinctive for her to ask herself, "How is this man feeling right now? Are his actions in line with how I think he feels? Are his words compatible with his body language and other facts?" So, a high-value woman is naturally empathetic, but she uses her empathy very consciously and does not let it be used against her.

Self-reliance

They are self-reliant, particularly in the emotional department. In other words, high-value women are fully in charge of their lives and their emotional well-being.

Self-reliance is a much bigger concept that goes beyond emotional mastery, but it has a huge emotional component. And the reason for that is that developing self-reliance is a road traveled alone, which triggers a range of negative emotions such as fear, anxiety, and pain. So, becoming self-reliant means, you have to first face those negative emotions and overcome them. Self-reliance also means you do not rely on external sources to feel good about yourself or to alter a negative emotional state. You do not rely on a partner to make you happy. You do not expect your friends to make you feel better. You don't even depend on material things such as new clothes, shoes, or a new bag to make you happy.

A high-value woman taps into her inner resources to alter her emotional state. She also recognizes when she's dependent on others for her well-being and works on diminishing that dependency. Self-reliance means you make your own decisions. You may seek other people's opinions or input, but the final decision is always yours. Sometimes you don't even tell other people about your dilemmas, which means you must rely on yourself, your judgment, and your inner compass to make the right decisions. Self-reliance also means you're thinking independently. A high-value woman relies on her reasoning and intuition to assess situations or develop her opinions and ideas.

The ability to think autonomously goes hand in hand with trusting your internal guide. Many people tend to hide behind what they've learned from society or other people within the society, which is symptomatic of their lack of confidence in their intuition and rational capabilities. Again, a high-value woman is self-reliant in that if she believes in something and considers that it holds merit after thinking it through, it becomes her truth, and she confidently voices it.

Finally, self-reliance also means you assume responsibility for everything in your life, even for things that are not your fault. Most people, when particularly uncomfortable with something, tend to find other people or other circumstances to blame. But high-value women are not looking to point fingers at anyone or anything, or at least they are not stuck there. For example, it may not be your fault to have been brought up in a toxic family and the psychological damage that it may have caused you, but it's your responsibility to change that damage that it caused you because it is yours, and if you don't take that responsibility, no one will.

In the context of relationships, most people quickly blame their partners for many things that go wrong in their life. But even when the wrongdoing of a partner is undeniable, for example, if the partner is cheating, a high-value man has the mindset of taking full responsibility for picking that person in the first place. Of course, this does not excuse any wrongdoings, but it prevents the high-value woman from losing her power to anyone else.

Don't take life too seriously

I know it is hard to achieve this because society has designed life so that everything is to be taken very seriously. Getting an education is a very serious matter, and making money and finding a life partner are very serious matters. But the truth is that at the end of it all is death – this should be a reminder not to take all of it too seriously beyond what is reasonable. Enjoy every step of the way with a little sense of lightweightness.

This used to be one of my biggest weaknesses, taking things too seriously, but now I have learned to be selectively serious, serious in my actions and my intentions, but not take it too seriously so that I always have a high degree of emotional detachment from outcomes. High-value women take few things to heart, and this attitude towards life allows them to have high degrees of emotional detachment and move in life with a lot of grace.

Chapter 9: Emotional Needs of Men that Make them Addicted to Women

Men live in an emotionless world most of the time. They don't get to feel and experience their emotions much outside of a romantic relationship. In this chapter, I will explain how tapping into the invisible world of emotions can make a man addicted to you and never think of leaving you. Specifically, I will tell you about four emotional needs you should try to meet if you want to keep a man in love with you over the long term.

Let's first talk about what attracts a man initially. Men are visual creatures first and foremost. They are attracted to how a woman looks and her physical attributes. There are evolutionary reasons for that as men must secure the best chances to pass on their genes. Therefore, they must select the most fertile and healthiest women they can get. It's programmed in their DNA to look for signs of good health and fertility, such as glowing skin, hair, body shape, etc.

After that initial stage of attraction, a man gets to know a woman on a deeper level, and that's when her personality, values, lifestyle, and other non-physical attributes come into play. But still, this isn't enough to keep a man around. We see that every day with people who are very much attracted to each other and who went through these two stages, spent months or even years together, and still ended up breaking up.

That's because there is one thing that all men need from a woman, which many women misunderstand about how men work. It has to do with the invisible world of emotions. As I said before, men live in emotionless environments most of the time, again due to evolutionary reasons. Nature selected men who could suppress their emotions to perform certain tasks that keep them alive, such as hunting to get food or protecting their families from imminent danger. Therefore, nature did not afford the luxury of being naturally attuned to their emotions for men.

Most men suppress their emotions subconsciously because it's coded in their DNA. The only way a man connects to his emotions is through a woman. That's also why we say that men fall in love emotionally, not logically or rationally. Men feel that they are in love, and they cannot pinpoint why they are in love. They fall in love because she made them feel a certain way, a significant difference between men and women.

Therefore, the little secret to keeping a man in a relationship with you is enabling him to connect to his emotional world by meeting his emotional needs that he's not even aware of. If a man can feel the right emotions in your presence, he will never leave you. That's a secret that took me a long time to uncover.

Let me tell you about a man's four most important emotional needs.

Firstly, a man needs to feel trusted. He needs to feel that his woman trusts his judgment and ability to make good decisions.

How can you meet this need?

By not constantly challenging every decision he makes. Of course, if it's an obvious mistake, you should prevent it. However, in other cases, you should refrain from challenging him and go with his decision, letting him bear the consequences. You could also show that you don't need to know all the decisions and can navigate life blindly with complete trust in him.

This doesn't have to apply only to big decisions. You could let him choose the next car you buy without interfering, for example. Lastly, try to avoid always getting involved in the thought process that leads to making a particular decision. You don't need to know all the parameters all the time.

Secondly, a man needs to feel respected. He needs to feel that his woman respects him because her respect weighs more than many others he can get. It also triggers an emotional reaction in him that his job or his colleague could never trigger. If he does not get this emotional need met by his woman, he will eventually leave her.

Thirdly, a man needs to feel valued by his woman. He needs to know that his woman sees the value in everything he provides and is well aware of the efforts and the hard work that he puts in. You can meet this emotional need by simply acknowledging his efforts and saying how much you value him and that you don't take it for granted. Also, try not to be too demanding and require more effort from him, as that would suggest you don't realize everything he's already doing.

Lastly, a man needs to feel competent. He may know intellectually that he is competent, but there is a difference between knowing something intellectually and feeling it. From his job, he gets rewarded for his competence through the money he receives and other forms of recognition from his peers. However, from his relationship, he wants to feel competent in his woman's eyes. He basically wants her validation. So, what you can do to meet this need is ask him for help and compliment him on his good work.

Chapter 10: How to Train Men to Respect You

When it comes to relationships, it's important to establish boundaries and communicate your expectations. Some people might think it's crazy to train a man like a dog, but the truth is, if you don't set clear boundaries and enforce them, you'll end up with a partner who takes you for granted and hurts your feelings.

It's also essential to love and respect yourself first before expecting anyone else to treat you the same way. Don't let other women tell you what's right or wrong in your relationship. You create the rules and decide what's acceptable or not. Other women might be putting up with something they don't like, and they might try to convince you that it's normal, but don't fall for that.

For instance, I once dated a guy who started scrolling through social media on his phone while we were in bed together. It was something that I was extremely against, and I made it clear to him. However, he did it again the next day, and this time, he even watched a video of a half-naked woman shaking her booty right in front of me. I was livid and knew I couldn't tolerate that kind of disrespect.

I didn't bother yelling or arguing with him. Instead, I showed my frustration and told him he didn't respect my time and that watching that kind of video in front of me was disrespectful. I grabbed my stuff and left, even though it was three in the morning. I would rather sleep outside naked than allow a man to treat me that way.

When I expressed my discomfort and left his place, he followed me outside in his boxers, begging me to return and promising it wouldn't happen again. But I didn't care. As a woman, I should create boundaries and not let a man dictate them. If a guy crosses my boundaries, it's done, and I won't waste my time on him. I know that there are men out there who will put up with even the craziest of boundaries, so if you can't respect mine, then you're not worth my time.

The point is, if you don't establish and enforce your boundaries, you'll end up with a partner who doesn't respect you. Don't let anyone convince you that you're crazy or overreacting. It's your relationship, and you deserve to be treated the way you want to be treated. Don't settle for less.

Some women might think I'm being unreasonable, but I know my worth and expect respect. I won't settle for less. I don't need to ask other men or women if I'm crazy because I trust my feelings. If a guy makes me feel like crap, I'm gone. I won't put up with someone who treats me poorly or disrespects my boundaries. Men shouldn't be able to walk all over us and treat us however they want just because they think we'll put up with it. We need to love ourselves and demand respect.

In the case of the guy I mentioned earlier, I didn't break things off completely, but I told him I needed space to think. During the few days that I didn't talk to him, I went out and enjoyed my life. I did the sports I loved, hung out with friends, and even flirted with other men. Meanwhile, he was constantly calling and messaging me, begging for me to come back. But I didn't cave in. I know there are men who respect me and are willing to do whatever it takes to make me happy.

So, ladies, don't let men dictate your boundaries or make you feel like you're crazy for standing up for yourself. You deserve respect; if someone can't give it to you, they're not worth your time. Love yourself enough to demand respect, and don't settle for anything less.

It's important to give your partner space when they need it. Allow them to reflect on their actions, think about their wrongdoings, and realize how much they value you. You should never tolerate being taken for granted, and while your partner is reflecting, take the opportunity to enjoy yourself with friends and remind yourself of your worth.

A woman who allows her partner to mistreat her is doing herself a disservice. Women hold significant power over men and leaving a mistreating partner can be just as effective as using that power to get what you want. Don't be afraid to set boundaries and demand respect.

Seeking advice from other women when your partner upsets you is not necessary. You should trust your feelings and set your boundaries. Love yourself and demand the treatment you deserve. Other women may be jealous of how well you're treated when you demand respect and set boundaries.

Confidence is vital when it comes to getting what you want from a partner. Trust your feelings, and don't hesitate to ask for what you want. If your partner can't give it to you, move on and find someone who will. If more women adopted this mindset, they would have fewer problems with men.

Remember, you can demand respect and set boundaries in your relationships. Love yourself, trust your instincts, and don't settle for less than you deserve.

No matter your appearance, there's no reason to put up with someone who makes fun of you. There's no excuse for anyone to treat you poorly; you deserve better than that.

Ladies, please remember that negative emotions like stress, sadness, and anger can lead to diseases and aging. Don't allow men to kill you with these negative emotions slowly. Learn to love yourself, stop caring what other people think, and create your own rules. If a man disrespects you, insults something you can't control, or doesn't respect your time, it should be enough to make you leave. Your happiness and sanity are more important than putting up with someone who doesn't treat you as special and replaceable.

If a man wants to test you and take advantage of you, leave and enjoy your life. Allow him to think about how he should have changed and become better for you. Don't let negative emotions take over your life. Set boundaries and love yourself.

Chapter 11: How to Find a Man that will Spoil You

Finding the right guy takes time and effort, but by following the guideline below, you'll find a man who values you and invests in your relationship.

The first step is to find a man who likes you more than you like him. Of course, this can be more difficult than it sounds, as some men are good at convincing women that they are in love when they really aren't. If get excited about a man only to be disappointed in the end, it may be because you're unable to detect these kinds of men.

The second step is to look for someone who doesn't intimidate you – you should not be afraid of losing him. The man you don't care about losing is the one you can easily demand to spoil you. You should feel confident enough to state your opinion, even if he disagrees. If you're afraid to ask him for things or to buy you gifts, it's likely because you like him more than he likes you. You should look for a man you don't like more than he likes you, so you can easily ask him for the things you want.

Focus on finding someone who values you and is willing to invest in the relationship. This means finding a guy who knows you're out of his league and feels lucky to be with you. If a man doesn't think he's lucky to have you, he won't feel the need to put effort into the relationship.

Avoid playing manipulative games. It's unhealthy to try to manipulate someone into liking you more, especially if you're not even sure you like them. Instead, focus on finding someone who accepts you for who you are and doesn't require any games to keep them interested.

Next, prioritize finding a man you can depend on for help when needed. This means looking for someone willing to go out of their way to assist you when you're in a tough spot. These guys will be there to fix your car at 3 a.m. or help you with household repairs. Avoid men who are all talk and no action or only provide small favors like buying you food.

Work on your appearance. It's important to take care of your hygiene and appearance and ensure you always look presentable. This doesn't mean that you need to wear designer clothes or have a lot of money to spend on your appearance. It means you must look your best and take pride in your appearance.

You should know what your limits are and communicate them to your partner. It's important to set boundaries and stick to them.

Have your own money. It's unattractive for a woman to depend on a man for everything. You should have your own money and be able to take care of yourself. This doesn't mean your partner can't help you, but you should be able to support yourself.

Find a nice guy. A nice guy who is genuine and predictable is the best kind of man. You don't need drama; a nice guy will make your life easier and more peaceful.

Find a man with money – he should be able to provide for himself and his family. Raising children is extremely difficult and can become even more challenging without a supportive partner.

Choosing a stable partner may not be as exciting as an unpredictable partner, but it's a smarter choice in the long run. Seeing other women suffer in unhappy relationships can serve as a reminder to choose wisely and not settle for less. Ultimately, being in a healthy and happy relationship with a partner who provides for you will be much more fulfilling than constantly searching for a man who will spend money on you without real commitment or love.

Chapter 12: Feminine Energy Morning Affirmations

These affirmations will help you to connect to your feminine energy and start your day with ease and flow. Read these affirmations early in the morning – when you're still in bed, when you're doing your hair or makeup, or when you're having your breakfast.

I start my day with ease and flow.

I embrace my femininity.

I am radiant.

I am present.

I love my feminine energy.

I am enough.

I trust my intuition.

I am full of life.

I love myself.

I don't chase; I attract.

It is safe for me to rest in my femininity.

Elva B. Fagan

I am balanced, happy, and fulfilled.

I honor myself.

I am magnetic.

It's okay for me to feel my emotions, all of them.

I love my body.

I radiate light.

I am creative.

I am sensual.

I am worthy.

I am connected to my feminine energy.

I love being a woman.

I am divine.

My energy exudes femininity.

I take care of myself physically, mentally, and spiritually.

I honor my body.

I am love.

Elva B. Fagan

I am serene.

I am soft and gentle.

I am my priority.

I am graceful.

I am beautiful.

I express my emotions freely.

I am so proud of the woman I am today.

I deserve everything that my heart desires.

Harnessing Your Dark Feminine Energy

I radiate feminine energy.

I start my day with ease and flow.

I embrace my femininity.

I am radiant.

I am present.

I love my feminine energy.

I trust my intuition.

I am full of life.

Elva B. Fagan

I love myself.

It is safe for me to rest in my femininity.

I am balanced, happy, and fulfilled.

I honor myself.

I am magnetic.

It's okay for me to feel my emotions, all of them.

I love my body.

I radiate light.

I am creative.

I am sensual.

I am worthy.

I am connected to my feminine energy.

I love being a woman.

I am divine.

My energy exudes femininity.

I take care of myself physically, mentally, and spiritually.

Elva B. Fagan

I honor my body.

I am love.

I am serene.

I am soft and gentle.

I am my priority.

I am graceful.

I am beautiful.

I express my emotions freely.

I am so proud of the woman I am today.

I deserve everything that my heart desires.

I radiate feminine energy.

Femme fatale affirmations to Boost your Confidence

Read these affirmations out loud for at least 30 days to reprogram your mind.

I stay calm and then act on the problems with a solution-oriented mindset.

The less I respond to negativity, the more peaceful my life becomes.

I am kind, and I can be ruthless when I need to be.

I put a spell on people.

I am dangerously hot. Nobody can compete with me but me.

When I walk into the room, people watch.

I elegantly take up space.

People regret leaving me, but then it will be too late.

There's this shine about me; I am unforgettable.

I am not arrogant; I am confident.

My come up will be the best sweet revenge.

My life is unfolding perfectly right now. There's no past; there's no future; there's only present.

People regret leaving me, but then it will be too late.

I am the fine feminine energy.

I am a feminine force of feminine being. I stay calm and then act on the problems with a solution-oriented mindset.

The less I respond to negativity, the more peaceful my life becomes.

Elva B. Fagan

I am kind, and I can be ruthless when I need to be.

There's this shine about me; I am unforgettable.

I am magnetic.

I am the fine feminine energy.

I am a feminine force of feminine being.

I stay calm and then act on the problems with a solution-oriented mindset.

The less I respond to negativity, the more peaceful my life becomes.

I am kind, and I can be ruthless when I need to be.

I put a spell on people. Nobody can compete with me but me.

When I walk into the room, people watch.

I elegantly take up space.

People regret leaving me, but then it will be too late.

Magnetic Femininity Affirmations

I have fun and fertile energy.

Elva B. Fagan

I have a mystic aura.

It is impossible to forget me.

I have a calm, cool alert.

I am intriguing.

I am elusive.

I am mysterious.

I am sensual.

I know how to use my feminine power.

My voice is deep and mysterious.

My eyes are deep.

I know how to captivate others.

I can always get what I want.

I know how to use my magnetism.

I make the most of my appearance.

I know that my magnetism is more than looks.

Everything about me is intoxicating.

Elva B. Fagan

I master the art of seduction.

I speak, move, and walk with cool elegance.

My clothes enhance my aura.

I only wear what makes me feel and look amazing.

I carry myself with confidence.

I always have good body posture.

I walk and talk with confidence.

I am aware of my body language.

I move in a sensual way.

The way I walk and talk is unforgettable.

My smile is mysterious.

I am irresistible.

I have amazing eye contact.

I smell heavenly.

I know exactly what to say and how to say it.

I am in charge of any situation.

Elva B. Fagan

I am calm, cool, and collected.

I am confident in myself.

I am in control of my emotions.

I am in control of my life.

I am powerful.

I am pure temptation.

I know my worth.

I am selected.

I am very hard to get.

I am a high-value woman.

I have high standards.

I am aware of my seductive power.

I am charismatic.

I exude strong femininity.

It is hard to resist me.

I am intoxicating.

Elva B. Fagan

I am passionate.

I am seductive.

I exude an electric aura.

I am self-assured.

I respect myself.

I have strong boundaries.

I am enigmatic.

I am a strong magnetic woman.

Anchor these affirmations by sitting up proud and strong and smiling at yourself.

Chapter 13: Psychology Tricks to Get What You Want Out of People

In this chapter, we will discuss some psychology tricks that are basic but not commonly known. These tricks are used by many people and can be very effective. These simple psychological tricks can be handy in everyday situations. Using them lets you make your life easier and get what you want from others. Just remember to use them responsibly and not to take advantage of others.

So, let's get started.

The first trick is pretending to be a bad liar, especially when dealing with men. You can tell a made-up story about how lying makes your hands shake, leading him to believe you're a bad liar. This way, it will be more effective when you do have to lie because he'll believe that you're telling the truth.

The second trick is that people hate giving out information but love correcting others. If you give someone incorrect information, they will want to correct you. This can be useful when you need information from someone but they're reluctant to give it to you. For example, if you need to file a complaint against a manager, but the person on the phone won't give you their name, you can call back and ask for the manager by the wrong name. The person who answers the phone will likely correct you and give you the correct name.

The third trick is to say the person's name when talking to them. This makes people feel more comfortable and attracted to you. It catches their attention and shows that you're paying attention to them. It's a simple trick but can be very effective.

The fourth trick is to play dumb. This doesn't mean you should act completely clueless, but rather that you should act like you don't know how to do something in certain situations. Allowing others to do the work for you can make your life easier.

Making someone feel good about themselves when they're around you can also increase their liking towards you. Letting someone talk about themselves and praising them can make them feel important and valued, making them want to be around you more.

Spending time with someone in person is also important for developing feelings of love toward them. Texting too much can decrease feelings of attraction, so it's better to focus on spending time together in person.

If you want to make someone think about you more sexually, you can try teasing them on Facetime. For example, you can pretend to change clothes in front of them, which can increase their thoughts of you in a sexual way. However, it's important to ensure both parties are comfortable with this behavior and always respect boundaries.

This trick is one that I have used often in toxic workplaces. I would compliment people behind their backs instead of engaging in workplace drama. By avoiding gossip and talking positively about people, others would hear about my compliments and begin liking me more. This trick is surprisingly effective and can be useful in many social situations.

This trick can be used on romantic partners when annoyed or upset with you. For example, if your partner is a car enthusiast, you can ask them a question about cars to get them talking. This will distract them from their negative feelings and refocus their attention on something they enjoy. They will often forget what they were upset about in the first place, and you can get back to your relationship as usual.

This trick is more of a fun tactic than a psychological one. It involves setting expectations low so that people are surprised when you exceed them. For example, if you act a little more stupid than you really are around your friends, they will be shocked when they learn about your academic and professional accomplishments. This can make you seem more interesting and attractive because you are unpredictable and mysterious.

These tricks are not manipulative or harmful when used correctly. They can be helpful tools for achieving certain outcomes and making social situations more enjoyable. However, it is important to use them ethically and with respect for others.

Social tricks for influence

Using phrases like "You're right" or "You're correct" can be effective. These phrases make the other person feel smart and validated, making them more willing to listen to you. In customer service, thanking customers for their patience can be more effective than apologizing for a delay or mistake. Shifting the focus to a positive trait the person has can diffuse tension and make them less likely to argue with you.

If you are arguing with someone, try starting with agreement instead of disagreement. Find common ground and acknowledge their perspective before stating your own. This can help create a more positive interaction and increase the likelihood of finding a resolution.

Hand something to someone when they're on the phone, as they're more likely to take it without asking questions. This can be useful when you need to delegate work or get someone to do something for you. For example, you could change the deadline on a work folder and hand it over to someone on the phone, so they'll be more likely to complete it on time. If they ask why you gave it to them, you can simply apologize and say you got distracted.

Act happy and excited whenever you see someone, even if they don't like you. This can confuse them at first, but eventually, they'll start to feel happier and more excited when they see you. For example, if you're used to walking into the office to silence and boring "good mornings," try changing things by acting excited to see everyone. Compliment their outfits, ask how they are, and show genuine interest in their lives. They might be confused at first, but eventually, they'll start to respond positively and act excited to see you.

Being nice to mean people is also important, as this can have surprising results. Even if someone is rude, try to respond with kindness and understanding. You never know what might be going on in their lives or why they're acting that way. For example, if someone sends you rude messages, respond with kindness and try to defuse the situation. They might surprise you by revealing their true intentions and apologizing for their behavior. Ultimately, being nice to mean people can be a great way to improve your relationships and make new friends.

A trick that works well, especially with narcissists, is telling them a story about someone with similar annoying traits to them. However, you should be subtle about it and twist the story so that they connect the dots. This will make them reflect on their behavior and hopefully improve it.

When we eat, our brain assumes that we're in a safe and calm place – this also applies to animals. So, if you're doing something that makes you nervous, chew gum or eat food while doing it. For instance, if you're taking a driving test, chew gum. Your brain will assume that you're safe, which will help calm you down.

If someone is angry with you, try to stay calm. They might get angrier initially, but eventually, they'll feel ashamed of themselves for being so angry while you remain calm. This is because the angry person will start doubting whether they should have been angry in the first place. Your calmness might even calm them down eventually. However, be aware that some manipulators also use this technique.

Avoid using "I think" or "I believe" in your conversations or writing. These words make you sound unsure and lack confidence. Most people cannot tell the difference between brilliance and confidence. If you seem confident, people will assume you know what you're talking about and follow you.

Tricks to influence people's behavior

One useful trick for motivating yourself to learn a new skill or tackle a task is to tell yourself that you will only work on it for five minutes. For example, if you have a history test coming up, convince yourself that you will sit down and study for just five minutes. You will often find that once you start, you'll want to continue and study properly. This strategy can also work for other tasks, such as doing dishes.

If someone is preoccupied and holding something, you can hold out your hand, and they will often give you whatever they are holding. This can be a useful trick, especially if you need to get someone's attention or distract them from something else they are doing.

When walking through a crowded area, try looking directly at where you are trying to go instead of making eye contact with people. This can signal to others that you have a clear direction, and they will often move out of your way to let you pass.

Pay attention to their body language if you approach two people at a party who are already engaged in conversation. They may not want to talk to you if their feet are not pointing toward you. It's best to respect their space and leave them alone.

Smiling can actually make you feel happier. If you force yourself to make a big smile, you will likely notice a boost in your mood. Another trick is to wait for the right moment to ask for permission or make a request, such as waiting for your mom to be on the phone before asking to go out with a friend.

When making a request of someone, avoid using the phrase "could you." Instead, use the word "please" and state your request clearly. This can make it harder for the person to say no and can result in a more positive response.

Try yawning if you suspect someone is staring at or checking you out. If they are also looking at you, they may yawn too. Another trick is to look at your watch or point to it, as the person may also instinctively check the time.

Finally, be aware of phrases that can make you feel insecure or doubtful, such as "I have no problem with you being here" or "I don't care what everyone else says; I think you're cool." These types of statements can often be backhanded compliments or passive-aggressive comments.

Chapter 14: Traits of Women Who Have Activated their Dark Feminine Energy

In this chapter, we will discuss dark feminine energy traits, so whenever you see these traits, you can know that dark feminine energy is present, activated, or embodied. These traits can be used as a guide on how to understand what dark feminine energy truly is. You can also use it to activate dark feminine energy within you.

Boundaries

A woman who has embodied her dark feminine energy understands the importance of certain boundaries. She also sets boundaries and maintains and enforces them. She has no fear or hesitation in certain situations because she understands the importance of it. It is vital to her present self and also her future self.

A healthy boundary can look like (and this is one of my boundaries) limiting the number of people entering your home. For me, my home is my sacred space. It's the only place in the world where I can be my vulnerable self. Not anyone and anybody can come into my home because of many reasons. My energy is perfect for me. Somebody else's energy might not be bad, but their energy might not be perfect for me. You just want to be careful with all the energies that come in and out of your home, your sacred space. Or even if they do come into your home, they don't come into every space of your home. So, at the very least, a room in your home is completely imprinted with just your energy. And so, you can truly be your true self in that.

Discernment

Another dark feminine energy trait is discernment. Because dark feminine energy allows a woman to create space to connect with herself, she understands herself more once she does that. Then she also has clarity of mind; because of that, she can see and feel things for what it is. This ability of discernment will allow her to avoid getting into situations she doesn't want.

And because she has nurtured a relationship with her intuition, she can pick up on things. And even sometimes, she's unable to put it into words or even convey it to another person so that they can understand. She just feels it in her guts, and she just follows it. She follows it blindly.

Has this ever happened to you where you just had a feeling in your gut you followed it blindly, and then weeks or months later, it turned out that you made the best decision?

Even then, you couldn't explain it to yourself; sometimes, you couldn't explain it to other people. You couldn't put it into words, but it's just a feeling you had. You followed it, and it turned out to be the right guidance that you chose to follow.

Discernment is a common dark feminine energy trait because she has nurtured a relationship with herself where she can clearly feel, decide, and see things for what they truly are, regardless of what it looks like on the side.

Creativity

Another common trait of a woman who has embodied and activated her dark feminine energy is creativity. From others looking at her, she seems to have it all, whether it's true or not. She knows how to create her reality because she's not scared to want what she wants; therefore, she's not scared to go after it and make it her reality.

Once you have activated your dark feminine energy, it enables you to have the mindset of, "I can have it all. I deserve to have it all. I am worthy. Why wouldn't I be? Why wouldn't I be? I'm a whole woman. I have a whole womb. I am the center of creation. Everything that's here inevitably came from a womb." All those buildings, cars, and people who thought about it came from a womb.

Dark feminine energy allows you to go inward, hence the word "dark." The dark feminine energy requires you to go within. Go into the dark, go inside, and understand yourself fully. Connect with yourself from the brain to the toe to the womb to the chest.

When a woman has activated her dark feminine energy, she can be powerful because she is in tune with herself. And in that moment of being in tune with her dark feminine energy, she disregards the noise outside. A lot of the narratives that we have in society are not true or not fully true. And it's just limiting beliefs that limit us in our lives. And so, a woman who has activated her dark feminine energy can live beyond the limiting beliefs. She's able to disregard it, and she's able to create the life that she truly wants.

Transformation

A woman who has activated her dark feminine energy understands the power and importance of transformation and rebirth. This trait encourages a woman to let go of what no longer serves her and allow the new to come in so that she can continue to expand.

For example, it's like a snake shedding its skin. A snake sheds its skin for its betterment, longevity, and well-being. We are evolving daily – we become a different version of ourselves every year, every month. And so, letting go is a requirement because we're constantly expanding and evolving. And a woman who has embodied her dark feminine energy understands this and is fearless in doing it.

Many women don't let go of things that no longer serve them and block the way for new and authentic to come in. A woman who has activated her dark feminine energy can let go and allow transformation and rebirth to occur without guilt. Because she understands that it's just a part of life, and it is necessary for the well-being and the longevity of her life, and inevitably will be beneficial to the people around her, the people in her life, her children, her family, and most importantly, herself.

Let go of things that no longer serve you.

Conclusion

A woman connected to her dark feminine energy knows herself, understands her desires, and receives them effortlessly. She exudes a magnetic energy that is impossible to ignore.

This transformative journey into the mysteries of dark feminine energy will not only shed light on the hidden aspects of the feminine but also guide you on a path to embracing and harnessing the power of the dark feminine. You'll learn how to work with the shadow aspects of the feminine to heal and transform yourself, reclaim your inner power, and unleash the full potential of the dark feminine energy.

Before I go, I would like to thank you for reading this book to the end.

Elva B. Fagan

I poured my heart and soul into this book, believing it would resonate with many readers. I would be honored if you could share your honest thoughts about this book in a REVIEW.

Your insights and critiques would be valuable feedback for me and help other readers discover this book.

Good luck!

Printed in Great Britain
by Amazon